Secrets of a Weight Loss Renegade

Shannon Hager

Copyright © 2018 Shannon
Hager

All rights reserved.
ISBN: 1722107448

DEDICATION

To my family-Mom, Dad, and Daniel, who have always supported me, and Kenneth McDonald.

Table of Contents

1-Beginnings

I was born on August 11, 1976 in San Diego, California. Both my parents are teachers, and I have a twin brother, Daniel, who is 10 minutes younger than me. My dad taught at the Department of Defense schools as a Special Education teacher. My mom stayed home with us, and then went back to school when we were 6 years old. She became a business teacher, then a guidance counselor. We moved to Holland when I was 5 years old. Daniel and I did almost everything together, since we moved around so much.

I was born with my left leg just a little shorter than the right leg. I had to wear braces on my legs for the first 11 years of my life. I walked with my knees bent, and both feet were positioned outwards as I walked. The only thing that made the whole ordeal a little less painful is that I was skinny, and could get around fairly easy.

I will say that even though I was skinny, I was tired all the time. That got old real quick. I had to sit down a lot too. But I was able to ride my bike, and Holland is great for having private bike paths, Riding my bike was a way to forget my troubles. It also helped build my physical strength and made me feel like I could do physical activities. It also gave me mental stamina, which would help me in the coming years.

2-Childhood

Because my dad was a great teacher, we got moved several times during our time in Europe.

We lived in Holland for 3 years, England for 1 year, and Germany for 2 years. Needless to say, during our time there I really got to know and love European cuisine. And I'm not talking about fancy fare. I've always enjoyed simple food. My mom cooked all our food, so there was never a lot of junk food in our pantry. I also never snacked in between meals.

Looking back, I was also a picky eater. If we went to the Friteur stand (French fry stand) and my brother Daniel put mayonnaise and otherthings I didn't like on the fries, I couldn't eat any of his fries. I always preferred my fries plain.

This was the 1980s, so there weren't a lot of diverse restaurant choices in European cities like there is today. It was either a Dutch/German restaurant, or McDonald's. In Germany, I had my old standby, schnitzel and french fries, which I would get whenever I had any doubts about the food.

Then I thought 'I blew it for the day, so I'm not going to eat anything else.' Then I would be half starving, half bloated from all the salt. It was a never ending cycle.

I was in South Dakota for graduate school in speech pathology. I loved the kids but didn't like all the paperwork. So to cure this I would go the Hy-Vee grocery store, and then get whatever junk food I wanted.

One favorite was Tofutti, an ice cream sandwich that is made from Tofu. Never mind that I can't stand to eat Tofu in its natural state. The only way I'll eat it is if it's fried. But I could down those Tofutti like there was no tomorrow. There were 6 in a box, so they were gone pretty fast.

I also didn't have a scale in my apartment. Since I never had a weight problem before, weighing myself was never a priority for me. But now I was starting to get too big to ignore it. I now had a double chin, and my breasts looked and felt like balloons ready to burst. It got to the point where I didn't like to look at myself in the mirror. But I still wasn't ready to do anything.

I also did a lot of physical activity as a child, whether it was playing in the field at the end of our neighborhood, bike riding, walking, or climbing a tree. I wanted to do it all and I did. This is also why when I did have a treat, I really didn't gain any weight.

Things changed when I started working at McDonald's when I was sixteen. This was my first job, and of course one of the perks was discounted food. If there was something to try, I went ahead and tried it. Chocolate milkshakes, Quarter Pounder with Cheese, large fries- I ate it all without a care in the world. Back then I still could. I think if I had to pay full price for the food, I probably wouldn't have bought it. Or I would have thought twice before buying it.

I started to gain weight toward the end of high school. I wasn't doing as much physical activity and I was eating more high fat, sugary foods. If I had to single out one culprit that put me on the path to weight gain, it was drinking Cokes and other sugary drinks. First I drank the regular Cokes, and then I switched to Diet, telling myself that Diet was better. I may have just as well inserted an IV line filled with sugar into my vein and left it in there permanently.

My next job was as a bagger at Vons, a grocery store chain in California. Here I would bag food and collect shopping carts, so I was still getting physical activity. By this point I started eating at an amazing Mexican restaurant, Lolita's. The place was always packed, and their prices were dirt cheap. At that time you could get 5 rolled tacos with guacamole, which I always got, along with rice.

I would go home, then sit down at the TV and eat my food. I could always finish what I was going to eat in about 30 min. It would be 30 min of complete bliss, and then I would get sleepy and sluggish. I went from about 130 lbs to 145 without any struggle. Pretty soon I had to start buying new clothes.

When I would go shopping and look in the mirror, I would tell myself that I didn't look too bad. A little chubby, yes, but I could hide it with some black clothes, preferably all black. Black and navy were my favorite colors. Little by little I started to get bigger overall. I started to hide, both from myself and others.

I graduated from San Diego State University, and then moved to Washington, D.C. for my first job. I didn't know how to cook a proper meal. I just microwaved everything, or got lots of pasta and bread. Carbs tend to stretch a little when you're on a limited budget.

I proceeded to gain more weight, and then decided to go to the University of South Dakota for graduate school. There I continued my habit of eating lots of carbs. I also discovered Utz, a Midwest brand of potato chips, which if you're a chip lover, is paradise. Just enough salt, but not too salty, just the right combination of salt and crunch. They had so many Flavors too! This is where I discovered Dill Pickle chips, in addition to my beloved Salt & Vinegar! I would go by the grocery store, buy a few bags of them, then go home to my apartment by myself, turn on the TV, then stuff myself for 30 min. before descending into a food coma.

I would then feel like a complete slug for the rest of the day, and I would feel guilty.

Then I got depressed and things got worse.

3-I Get Depressed

I wasn't doing well in my clinical practicum. So to cope I ate more, didn't exercise, and didn't do much of anything else. Not having any family members in the area for support also didn't help. My family was 1500 miles away. For anyone to get to me took at least 2 days.

One night I felt so overwhelmed that I thought about harming myself. I hadn't ever felt that way before and didn't know what to do, so I went to the local hospital and told them I needed help.

I was then given a checklist by a nurse practitioner and told that I was depressed. I told her that I respected her, but wanted to see a doctor. I was then given a prescription for Xanax and told to come back.

The next day I made the mistake of taking a whole Xanax. It calmed me down within 10 minutes of taking it, but then it also knocked me out for 4 hours. I didn't want to be totally out of commission!

I went back to the doctor a day or two later. I told him what was going on-he gave me a prescription for Zoloft (I forget how many milligrams I was prescribed) and had me make a follow up appointment. He was a nice doctor and seemed willing to want to help me, which was what I needed.

I start taking the Zoloft and was told that the effects of it would take a couple of weeks to kick in. After about 3 weeks of taking it, I started to sweat very easily, which I could tolerate.

What I couldn't tolerate was insomnia, which is the most horrible condition to have. I would get tired, but no matter what I did I couldn't go to sleep at night. I never had trouble falling or staying asleep before. I could stay up all night, then when I would have to go to clinic I would start to feel tired and then I couldn't think clearly. It was the worst situation to be in.

Another side effect of the Zoloft was that it stimulated my appetite. I couldn't turn off my urge to eat; I was never satisfied. Some folks on Zoloft experience no desire to eat; that wasn't my case. So before I know it, I had ballooned up to

172 lbs. I had joined a weight loss group at the hospital and got weighed there, that was how I found out. I was so disgusted with myself. So I joined Weight Watchers for the first time in 2004.

4- First Round At Weight Watchers

I can tell you that the first time I joined Weight Watchers in South Dakota, I really wasn't ready to lose weight. I was disgusted with my body but not ready to change my eating habits.

The meetings were held in a church, and the leader provided good solid advice. Still, she didn't motivate me. I was still going to the Hy-Vee and getting Tofutti, and I was also buying frozen Weight Watcher meals and eating them after the meetings.

I was also still drinking Diet Cokes, and not drinking enough water. My favorite was Diet Coke with Lime. Once I started one of those, I easily went through 5-6 in a day. I also found that once I started drinking the Cokes, it acted as an appetite stimulant, so I could continuously graze on snacks all day.

I probably would have made some progress if I would have just increased my water intake.

But I wasn't ready to do that either. I just kept on drinking sodas like they were going out of fashion.I ended up leaving South Dakota at 175 pounds. But one thing I did take with me was my measuring spoons, just in case I would ever use them.

5- 2nd round at Weight Watchers

In 2011, I joined Weight Watchers for the 2nd and last time. My brother was getting married, so I wanted to look good. My mom and I joined together. My mom is 5-6 inches taller than I am. She looked better than I did, although we were both overweight.

I want to say that by this point, I was 36 years old and at that point had been fat for 12 years. As I got bigger and bigger I somehow told myself I didn't look that bad. I also never weighed myself, so I had no idea how out of control it had gotten. Somehow when you're overweight and you're out and about you notice the folks that are really overweight and you say to yourself, "Well, at least I'm not that bad off." That's what I would tell myself.

When I got weighed in for the first time, I was 175 pounds. I hadn't weighed myself in a while. All the same, it was still a shock. I will say that I went to the meetings for 1 year without losing any weight.

During this period, I still hadn't changed

my eating habits. I also wasn't exercising either.One thing I couldn't give up was iced coffee with cream and sugar. I figured out how to make my own coffee, and then got the flavored creamers I liked. I saved a lot of money doing this. I don't even go to Starbucks anymore.

In the first month, I lost 8 lbs. This was a great start. I didn't know anyone who had lost a lot of weight, so starting out I didn't have anyone to go to. But once I lost the first 10 pounds, I thought "I can do this!"

It took me 6 months to lose the first 20 lbs. By then my clothes were so big I had to get new ones. I tried to wait as long as I could before spending a lot of money on new clothes.

It took another year and 4 months before I got down to 120 pounds, my personal target weight. This is the weight where I feel my best, and I feel that wanting to be a particular weight is a really personal decision. This should be discussed with a doctor if there are any other questions or if one has any medical conditions.

Exercise is another area that is crucial in the weight loss journey. If you don't exercise, you can still lose weight, but the weight loss will be slower. At the beginning of my journey I didn't exercise at all. I started exercising 2-3 times a week. I figured that was a good start. Some weeks I exercised more, sometimes less.

Another thing that Weight Watchers teaches you is to eliminate all chicken, fish, etc. with any type of breading on it.I would exercise, then make myself a sandwich with breaded chicken. Another tip is to try to reduce carbs, such as lot of rice or bread. I was also at this point still eating a lot of carb-rich foods, like bread and pasta.

I also wasn't drinking enough water. It seems like such an easy, intuitive concept-drink lots of water!! But when you're so used to drinking lots of coffee and coke, it's hard to drink water.

Somehow, I had told myself that I was the exception. I didn't need to follow any rules. But I was really kicking myself in the foot and wasting time.

Then one week the leader challenged us to write everything down for just 1 week and see if it made a difference. I decided to do it. I bought myself a journal and wrote everything down. Having to do this made me more conscious of what I was actually eating.

Trust me, if you don't write things down, you

will never remember what you ate that day or week. I thought I could remember, but when I would get weighed and there was no change, or a gain, no one could give me any feedback. So writing in a journal was very helpful for me.

I would recommend doing some physical activity at least 2-3 times a week to start. It doesn't have to be Tae Bo or anything like that. Picking an activity you enjoy is the best way to bring fitness into your life. You will look forward to doing it, and it won't seem like a chore.

I want to point out that I am still on my weight loss journey. I have to take it one day at a time, one meal at a time. I still write everything down in my food journal. Some weeks are good, some are bad. Keep pushing on and stay positive!

6- My Favorite Recipes

French Lentil & Goat Cheese Salad with Dill

Serves 4

This recipe comes from the Weight Watchers Points Plus Power Foods Cookbook

<u>Ingredients:</u>

6 cups water
1 cup green (French) lentils, picked over, rinsed, and drained (or any other kind of lentils)
¾ teaspoon salt
2 celery stalks, diced
2 carrots, cut into matchstick-thin strips 1 shallot, minced
3 tablespoons white wine vinegar 2 tablespoons minced fresh dill
1 tablespoon olive oil
1 tablespoon Dijon mustard
½ teaspoon black pepper
3 ounces goat cheese, crumbled

1. 1.Bring water, lentils, and ½ teaspoon salt to boil in large saucepan.Reduce heat and simmer uncovered, until lentils are tender but hold their shape, 15-20 minutes. Drain; transfer to large bowl to cool.Add celery, carrots, shallot, vinegar, dill, oil, mustard, pepper, and remaining ¼ teaspoon salt to lentils and stir to combine Stir in goat cheese just before serving. Serve chilled or at room temperature.

Per serving (1 ½ cups): 263 calories, 9g total fat, 4g sat fat, 0g trans fat, 10 mg Chol, 676 mg Sodium, 33g Carb, 3g Sugar, 8g Fiber, 14g Protein, 86mg Calc.
Weight Watchers Points Plus Value: 7

Note: This salad is a staple of mine. It's not too hard to make; the only time intensive tasks are cutting up the veggies. If you're not sharing the salad with anyone else in your home, this salad yields a huge portion that you can eat throughout the week. I liked this salad because it didn't leave me feeling bloated, and filled me up until the next meal.

I also like this salad because it gives me an option to go vegetarian. Going vegan in my experience is both easier on the waistline a wallet. If you have to throw out some of the salad because you couldn't eat it fast enough, or find that you don't like it, you won't feel too guilty.

You can eat this lentil salad either with the goat cheese or without it. You can also add more veggies to it, such as bell peppers and cucumbers. This is the perfect refreshing salad for the summer or anytime!

Chicken Fried Rice
Serves 4 Under 20 minutes
From the Weight Watchers Points Plus Power Foods Cookbook

Ingredients

1 tablespoon tomato paste
1 tablespoon Asian fish sauce-optional-I don't use this ingredient-it makes it taste too fishy for me
3 teaspoons canola oil

2 large eggs, lightly beaten
3 scallions, thinly sliced
2 garlic cloves, minced
2 teaspoons minced peeled fresh ginger
1 1/2cups diced cooked skinless chicken breast
1 (8.8-ounce) package cooked brown
   rice (about 1 ¾ cups)
2 plum tomatoes, chopped (you can also use
grape tomatoes)
2   tablespoons chopped fresh cilantro

1. Whisk together tomato paste and fish sauce in small bowl until smooth; set aside.
2. Heat large heavy skillet or work over medium heat until a drop of water sizzles in pan. Add 2 teaspoon of oil and swirl to coat pan. Add eggs. Stir-fry until firm, about 2 minutes. Transfer scrambled eggs to plate.
3. Heat remaining 2 teaspoons oil in same skillet. Add scallions, garlic, and ginger and stir-fry until softened, about 3 minutes. Add chicken and rice; stir-fry until rice is coated, about 1 minute. Add tomatoes and tomato paste mixture; stir-fry until tomatoes are softened, about 2 minutes. Remove from heat, stir in eggs

and cilantro. Serve at once.

Per serving (1 cup): 240 calories, 8g Total Fat, 2g Sat Fat, 0g trans fat, 152 mg Chol, 455 mg sodium, 19g carb, 2g sugar, 2g fiber, 22g protein, 42mg calcium. Weight Watchers Points Plus Value: 6

Note: This recipe is great for the whole family- my whole family has it, and it's a hit! You can also substitute cooked shrimp. I like to make a large batch, and portion it out into individual bags and freeze them. Then I can pull them out of the freezer as I need them. I can't tell you how many times this recipe has saved me from diving into the potato chips or crackers!

Devil's Food Cupcakes with White Icing Squiggles
Makes 12
From the Weight Watchers Points Plus Best Darn Food Ever! Cookbook

<u>Ingredients:</u>

1 cup cake flour
¾ cup sugar
½ cup unsweetened cocoa
1 ounce semisweet chocolate, grated 2 teaspoons instant expresso powder 1 teaspoon baking powder
½ teaspoon salt
¼ teaspoon baking soda 1 large egg
1 egg white
½ cup fat free milk
½ cup fat free sour cream
¼ cup canola oil
1 teaspoon vanilla

extract Glaze:

½ cup dark or semisweet chocolate chips
¼ cup fat free milk
White decorative icing

1. Preheat oven to 375 degrees. Spray 12-cup muffin pan with nonstick spray.
2. To make cupcakes, whisk together flour, sugar, cocoa, grated chocolate, expresso powder, baking powder, salt, & baking soda in medium bowl. Whisk together egg, egg white, milk, sour cream, oil, and vanilla in small bowl. Add milk mixture to flour mixture, stirring just until blended.
3. Fill prepared muffin cups about 2/3 full with batter. Bake until toothpick inserted into center of cupcake comes out clean, about 25 minutes. Let cool in pan on wire rack, 10 minutes. Remove cupcakes from pan and let completely cool on rack.
4. To make glaze, place chocolate chips and milk in small microwavable bowl. Microwave on high 30 seconds, stir. Microwave until chocolate is melted and mixture is smooth, 10-15 seconds longer. Let stand 10 minutes to cool and thicken slightly.
5. Dip tops of cupcakes into glaze, turning to coat. Let cupcakes cool on rack until glaze is set, about 20 minutes. Pipe little circles of icing in lines across tops of cupcakes.Per serving (1 cupcake): 203 calories, 9 g total fat, 3g sat fat,

0g trans fat, 19 mg chol, 202 mg sodium, 30g carb, 17g sugar, 2g fiber, 4g protein, 49mg calc. Weight Watchers Points Plus Value: 6. These cupcakes look and taste like the Hostess cupcakes, and with a lot less calories and fat!

Cilantro Pesto-Grilled Vegetables and Pasta
Serves 4 plus leftovers
From the Weight Watchers Points Plus I Love Leftovers Cookbook

<u>Ingredients:</u>

2 red bell peppers, quartered lengthwise
2 large yellow squash, cut lengthwise into thick slices
2 large zucchini, cut lengthwise into thick slices
1 large red onion, cut into ¼ inch slices
8 ounces whole wheat spaghetti
¼ cup prepared cilantro or basil pesto sauce
¼ cup reduced sodium chicken broth
¼ cup reduced fat feta cheese

1. Spray grill rack with nonstick spray and prepare medium-hot fire.
2. Place bell peppers, yellow squash, zucchini, and onion in large bowl; lightly spray with nonstick spray. Place vegetables on grill rack and grill, turning often, until lightly browned and crisp-tender, 8-10 minutes. Transfer to cutting board; cut into 1-inch pieces. Transfer 2 cups of grilled vegetables

to container and let cool.

3. Cook pasta according to package direction; transfer to large serving bowl. Add reserved vegetables, pesto, and broth, toss to combine. Sprinkle with feta cheese.

Per serving (1 ¾ cup pasta mixture and 1 tablespoon cheese): 335 calories, 9 g total fat, 2g sat fat, 0g trans fat, 8mg chol, 273 mg sodium, 53 g carb, 8g sugar, 11 g fiber, 15g protein, 116 mg calc. Weight Watchers Points PlusValue: 9

This is a great dish that makes for eating all week!

German Potato Salad with Bacon and Red Onion
Serves 4
From the Weight Watchers All-American Comfort Cookbook

<u>Ingredients:</u>

1 ½ pounds small Yukon Gold potatoes, scrubbed
4 slices turkey bacon, cut crosswise into ¼ inch matchstick strips
1 teaspoon canola oil
1 small red onion, finely chopped
¼ cup reduced sodium chicken broth
2 tablespoons unseasoned rice vinegar
2 tablespoons finely chopped fresh flat-leaf parsley
1 tablespoon snipped fresh dill
¼ teaspoon salt
¼ teaspoon black pepper

1. Put potatoes in large saucepan with enough cold water to cover; bring to boil. Reduce heat and simmer until potatoes are tender, about 15 minutes. Drain potatoes in

colander and let cool until just cool enough to handle.

2. Cook bacon in medium nonstick skillet until crisp. Drain on paper towels and crumble. Measure bacon drippings; add enough oil to equal 2 teaspoons. Set aside.

3. Slip skins off potatoes. Cut potatoes in quarters. Transfer to medium bowl and keep warm.

4. To make dressing, heat drippings with oil in same skillet over medium heat. Add onion and cook, stirring frequently until softened, about 4 minutes. Stir in broth and vinegar, bring to simmer. Pour hot dressing over potatoes, add bacon, parsley, dill, salt, and pepper, toss gently until mixed well. Let stand until some dressing is absorbed, about 2-3 minutes. Serve warm, at room temperature, or cold.

Per serving (1 cup): 202 calories, 5g total fat, 0g trans fat, 14 mg chol, 517 mg sodium, 32g carb, 3g sugar, 4g fiber, 7g protein, 46 mg calc. Weight Watchers Points Plus Value: 5

This is a great comfort dish when you just want a big heap of potatoes!

Spaghetti with Mushrooms, Asparagus, & Dill
Serves 4
From Weight Watchers 360 Family Style

Ingredients:

6   ounces whole wheat spaghetti
1 bunch asparagus, trimmed and cut into 1 ½ inch pieces
2   teaspoons olive oil
3   shallots, thinly sliced
¾ pound mixed wild mushrooms
½ teaspoon salt
  2 teaspoons all purpose flour
1 cup reduced sodium chicken or vegetable broth
¼ cup fat free half and half
  3 tablespoons chopped fresh dill
  4 tablespoons grated reduced-fat Parmesan cheese

1. Cook pasta according to package directions. Add asparagus during last 3 minutes of cooking. Drain.
2. Heat oil in large skillet over medium-high heat. Add shallots and garlic and cook, stirring often, until shallots soften, about 2-

3 minutes. Add mushrooms and salt, stirring often, until liquid thickens slightly, about 3 minutes. Add half and half and cook until heated through. Add pasta with asparagus, dill, and 2 tablespoons Parmesan, toss to coat.

Per Serving (1 ¼ cup pasta and 1 tablespoon Parmesan): 262 calories, 4g total fat, 1g sat fat, 0g trans fat, 4mg chol, 409 mg sodium, 46g carb, 7g sugar, 8g fiber, 15g protein, 140mg Calc. Weight Watchers Points Plus Value: 7.

ABOUT THE AUTHOR

Shannon Hager is taking her weight loss journey one day at a time. She lives in North Carolina. When not reading or writing, she enjoys spending time with her family. She has an M.A. from the University of South Dakota.

www.ingramcontent.com/pod-product-compliance
Lightning Source LLC
Chambersburg PA
CBHW070102260726
48658CB00002B/960